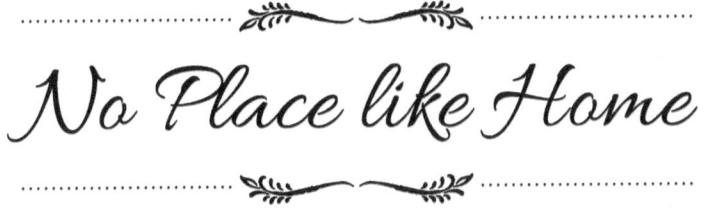

No Place like Home

An Organized Reference Guide to Caring for a Friend or Loved One at Home

Joyce Greene

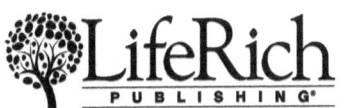

LifeRich Publishing is a registered trademark of
The Reader's Digest Association, Inc.

LifeRich Publishing books may be ordered through booksellers or by contacting:

LifeRich Publishing
1663 Liberty Drive
Bloomington, IN 47403
www.liferichpublishing.com
1 (888) 238-8637

Because of the dynamic nature of the Internet, any web addresses or
links contained in this book may have changed since publication and
may no longer be valid. The views expressed in this work are solely those
of the author and do not necessarily reflect the views of the publisher,
and the publisher hereby disclaims any responsibility for them.

The author of this book does not dispense medical or financial advice or
prescribe the use of any technique as a form of treatment for physical,
emotional, medical or financial problems without the advice of a
physician and /or financial professional, either directly or indirectly. The
intent of the author is only to offer information of a general nature to
guide you. In the event you use any of the information in this book, the
author & the publisher assume no responsibility for your actions.

Interior Images by Dreamstime.com and Pond5.com

ISBN: 978-1-4897-0617-1 (sc)
ISBN: 978-1-4897-0618-8 (e)

Library of Congress Control Number: 2015919684

Print information available on the last page.

LifeRich Publishing rev. date: 2/4/2016

For

My Mother, Louise, all of her dedicated caregivers, my family and of course, my husband David and my other Mother, Fran Greene. I love you all!

Contents

Acknowledgements

Thanks to my Father, Vince, who was always my biggest fan. He was a great storyteller and I listened carefully to each and every one he told. I remembered them all in such great detail, and cherish his memory!

Thanks to my Mother, Louise, for instilling the compassion in me, and caregiving ability which led me to this knowledge and ultimately, this book. She gave me the opportunity to take great care of her while getting the education of a lifetime.

Thanks to my other mother, Fran Greene, who actually pushed me to write about my life and caregiving. She and my other father, Herb, have truly been a guiding source of encouragement and love! I miss him dearly.

Thanks to my brother, Vince, my lifelong confidant, for his constant love and encouragement to pursue my goals! Thanks to my baby brother Rick for his arrival in my life. He inspires me with nourishment and love, and motivates me to reach for the stars! They are always by my side, and continue to be my lifeline as the years go by.

Thanks to my brilliant daughter, Amy, who was a constant supporter and my main editor in assisting me to write this book. Her uplifting spirit and dedication enabled me to finally finish my book! She and her husband Jeff have given us our beautiful grandchildren, Ashlyn, Jeffrey and Ethan, who light up our lives. Also, thanks to my sisters Carol and Susan and brother-in-law, Michael for their love. They have given me my incredible nieces & nephews, Alex, Max, Alena & Julia, and have allowed me a close place in their lives. I love them madly.

Thanks to my niece, Liz, whom I consider more of a daughter than a niece! She and her family, Brad, Shelby & Woods are examples of her spiritual nature and innate goodness. Thanks to my Aunt Mary and Uncle George, who kept me by their side as a child, with Georgette, my favorite childhood partner in crime, and considered me a part of their family. They gave me unconditional love and support which inspired me throughout my adult life.

Thanks to my extended family, The Lumnica's & Gjocaj's, for allowing me to be a part of Xhemile's life, a true angel, whom I love dearly. Also thanks to Elida, my sister and best friend, Tim and their amazing children, Glorida, Elvis and Sonila, who have always loved me as their family. Thank you for sharing them.

Thanks to my special friend, Marguerite, who has filled so many voids in my life by allowing me into hers. She has taught me many lessons and has been a constant source of education and has enabled me to feel true gratitude and love for her.

Thanks to my lifelong friend, Marilyn, for her never-ending friendship! I cherish our wonderful memories we've shared throughout our lives.

Thanks to my longtime friend, Ernest, for being the funniest guy I know. Our life episodes go beyond amazing. Erne', you are so talented!

Thanks to my amazing healer, Joann, who has been a loving friend, as well. Your energy and nurturing will remain with me in this life & the next.

Thanks to my amazing massage therapist, Carlene, for keeping me relaxed and balanced. Her calming demeanor is like no other.

Thanks to Denise, my friend and "right arm" for a million years…for her friendship and loyalty in our business, and making it possible for me to concentrate on my book. Thank you Glorida & Sonila for being my personal assistants and joy in my life. And thanks to Shawn & my staff for their hard work & loyalty.

Thanks to the many doctors, nurses, administrators and caregivers who helped contribute to my knowledge and understanding of medicine, and how it relates to the elderly.

And of course, special thanks to my wonderful life partner, David. The stars definitely aligned when we met! You are my shoulder when I need one, and my biggest supporter and best friend...I love you always...ywfl

Introduction

For most of us, caring for our parents or spouses can be a very difficult decision and time consuming endeavor.

I began caring for many family members as a young child, learning simply by being present. I quickly found that care and nurturing were the most important elements in the healing process, and helped invaluably in the transition from this life to the next.

Being a natural caregiver on so many levels, I always knew I could make this gift one which could live on through me. Now, I am caring for my mother, the person who was my first teacher. I have expanded on these caregiving qualities, and I intend to share many of my ideas, and knowledge in this reference guide. Through doing so, you, too, will be capable of organizing and caring for your loved ones to the best of your ability!

CHAPTER 1

Advocates

Advocates for non-medical assistance can be utilized in many ways, such as: volunteers, family members, live-ins, & full or part-time aides. The need must be determined by family or professionals, according to patient's health and independence.

Once the decision has been made to begin plan of care, ads and word of mouth are excellent steps to locate caregivers. I have always asked staff in doctor's offices, and aides and nurses in hospitals or nursing home facilities.

Interviews and references are a must. Once hired, training is very important. Every patient is an individual case, and should be carefully matched with advocates and caregivers. In this process, someone should decide who will be the main advocate for the particular patient. This person will be responsible for the overall system about to be created.

Once the person is chosen, the hiring begins, as does the scheduling and time periods for each shift. I usually set up large calendars in the kitchen area, where all aides, therapists, appointments, etc. are logged. Everyone signs in and the main person in charge will pay all advocates and helpers. It is also helpful for notating therapists, Dr. appointments, etc. on this main calendar in chapter #3.

The main function of the aides is to help make the patient feel safe and comfortable. I usually use alternative therapies to relieve pain, such as heat packs and keep them healthy, while raising immunities. I have many dietary ideas that are mentioned in another chapter #5. All aides are trained for individual's needs and preferences.

It is also necessary to plan for the caregiver's health & well- being as well. If they are happy & healthy, they perform better. Being with the patient day after day is very trying and can take its toll on anyone. There are many support groups available to help comfort and counsel for optimum benefits.

CHAPTER 2

Safety

Safety is probably the most important issue to approach! Helping the patient remain in their home safely is our priority. Accessibility with ramps, space for wheelchairs and walkers can enable them to become a little more independent, as well as canes,

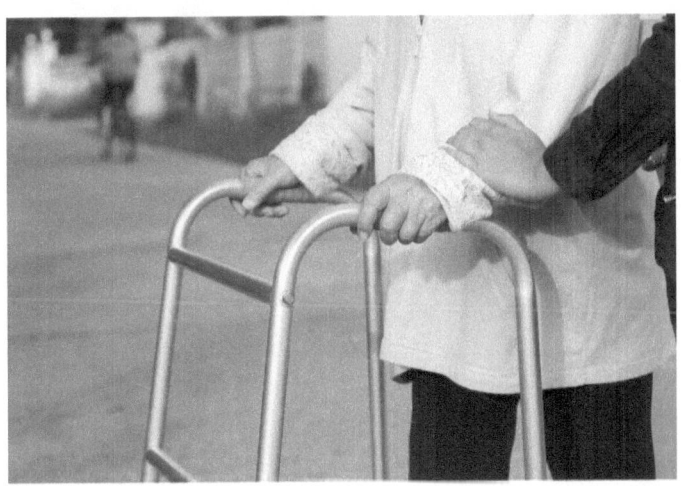

walkers, etc. These items can be found in pharmacies, on amazon.com, ebay.com, or generally google searching what you are looking for.

Steps and walkways should be in good condition, with rails and treads for gripping. No layering of carpets on carpets to eliminate tripping. Also, lighting is so important for the elderly.

Bathrooms are often very dangerous spaces for someone with balance and weakness conditions. Always have shower chairs and bars installed, in addition to commodes in order to raise toilet seats for easier on and off. Remove all mats on floors to eliminate accidents as far as tripping, and falling. If patient is a fall risk, the aide should stay with patient at all times.

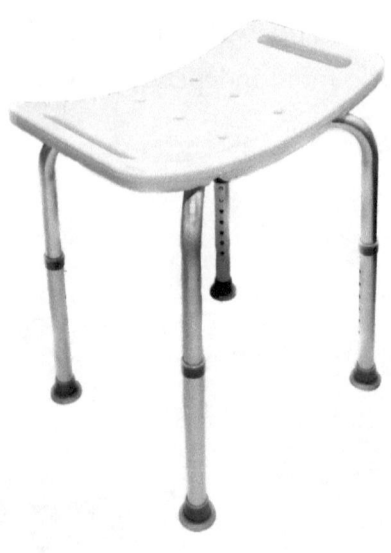

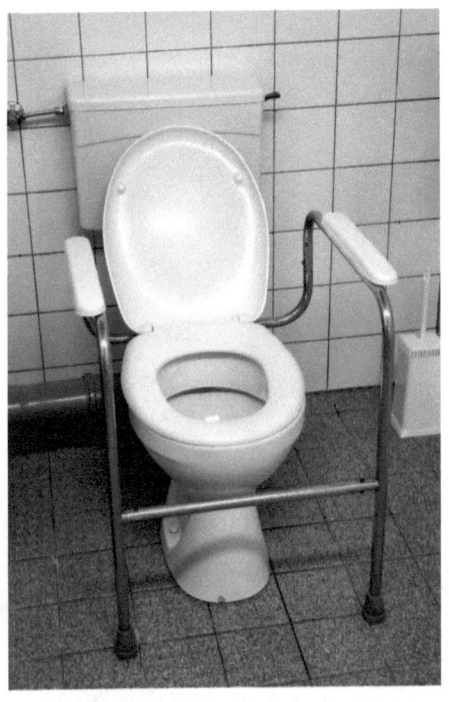

Bedrails are helpful in lifting the patient in and out of bed. The best solution is a motorized bed, raising head, back & or legs. It is ideal to leave a commode in the bedroom next to the bed so the patient does not have to walk unassisted in the night. Electric recliners are very comfortable and easily bring patients to a standing position, who are experiencing back weakness and pain. "La-Z-Boy" is a popular recliner brand, which can be previewed online, and your local retailer can be found online, as well.

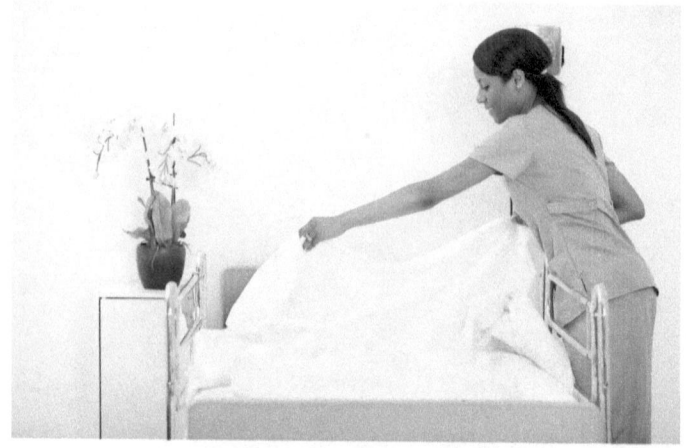

"Life Alert" and "First Alert" are reassuring for our loved ones- the system is inexpensive for the peace of mind you receive. An emergency box is centrally located and if alarm is set off, a live person speaks to the patient and remains on the line until help arrives. They also include a necklace with an emergency button.

An extra house key should be given to at least one caregiver so access to the home is possible at all times. In addition to the obvious safety features, smoke alarms, flashlights, night lights and lanterns are so important. Check for batteries, and consider a fire extinguisher in the kitchen area.

Dead bolt locks on all doors are usually the best way to secure safety for all in the home. Always keep doors locked after entering, train caregivers not to let anyone in unless a prior plan has been made.

Safety is also essential for the caregiver. Upon entering the home, caregiver should immediately WASH HANDS. The caregiver should also be using masks and gloves when necessary. For example: emptying dishwasher, preparing food, bathing, and cleaning the home. When caregivers are conscientious, the patient can remain healthier and feel the respect they deserve.

Another helpful idea is to utilize baby monitors, which are especially wonderful assets for family members or caregivers that are sleeping over. It's comforting for our patient to know if they need help, there is someone listening!

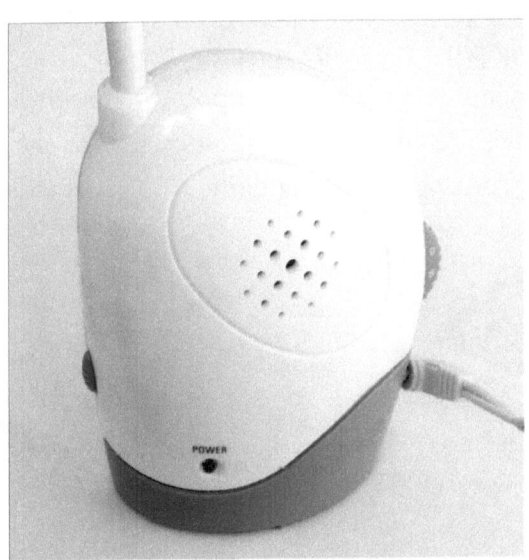

CHAPTER 3

Organizing the home

Organizing the home is so important. Copies of a health history should be on file and medical records are a big plus- the more info, the better.

Calendars for events, appointments, and aides schedules are always helpful, especially for the many people coming and going daily.

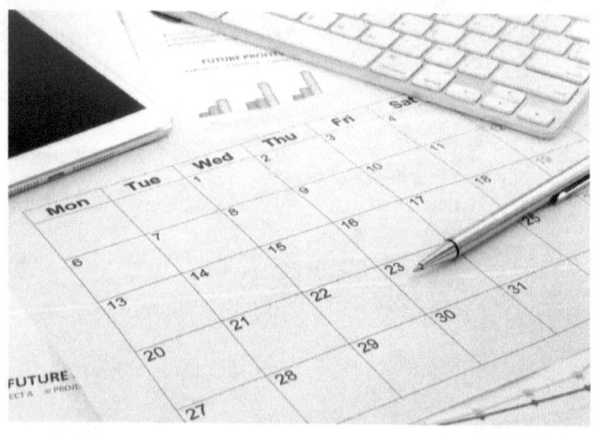

This is a great place to list family & worker's numbers to be available for all to see.

I always have lists of current drugs posted, as well as an organized and personalized dry erase board, where I notate exercise, fluids, meds taken, meals, etc. This is a great way to avoid mistakes and for everyone to be informed.

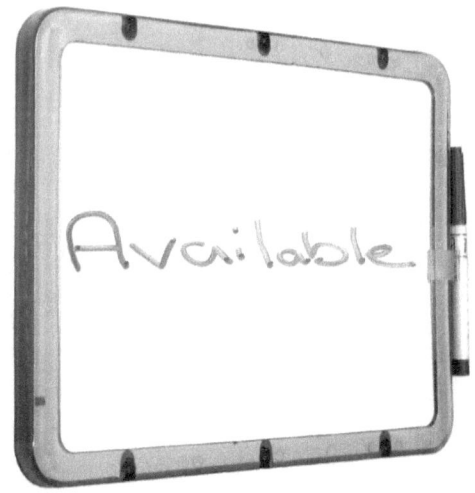

I usually purchase dry-erase calendars and boards online or in "Staples". It makes it very easy to make changes daily, while keeping certain information in permanent markers that remains month to month. There are photos you may utilize for reference.

Pads for to do lists are a good way for caregivers to stay efficient and to coordinate the day and many necessary chores.

It is important to know how to care for the home, whether they are in an apartment or in their own home. A list of superintendant, neighbors, gardeners, heating & electric companies, cable, phone, plumbers etc. are essential.

I have incorporated examples of lists in the back of this guide for your convenience.

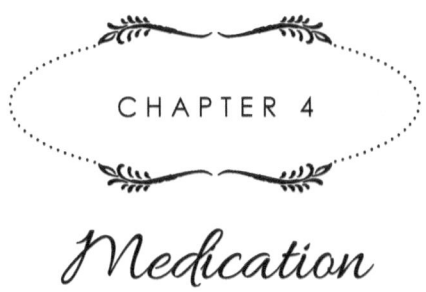

CHAPTER 4

Medication

It is important for any/all caregivers to be well-informed about what medications the patient is currently taking. The caregiver should contact a local pharmacy in order to tap into important info such as drug safety, and interaction. You will need to use a pharmacy which delivers. Create an index card with all times given and names of drugs, plus allergies.

Use a **PILL BOX,** which has slots for seven days, with morning, lunch, dinner and bedtime. Keep track of drugs on your board. This is an essential part of keeping patients safe. In the event that patients cannot swallow pills, verify if meds can be crushed, and obtain a pill crusher or mortar and pestle and mix in applesauce or yogurt.

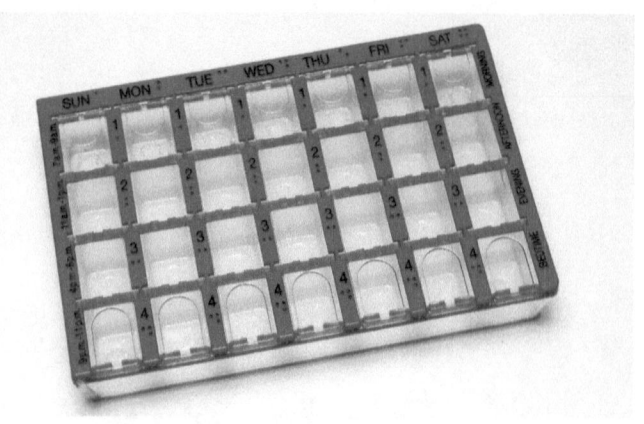

Always consider the importance of medications, therefore you need to make it possible to administer at all times. Make one person in charge of filling the pill box, and keep track of refill dates. Ask pharmacy to refill automatically, so you will not be in a position to run out of anything!

Pharmacists are very knowledgeable and should be contacted with any questions as far as the patient's medications. Never hesitate to ask, as special precautions should be taken with any controlled substances to avoid overdose or abuse.

Some important over the counter (OTC) items that are beneficial to keep on hand are:

Vitamins: "Vitamelts" dissolve in mouth, some general recommendations would be: vitamin D, B12 for energy, vitamin C to boost immune system

OTC pain meds (ie: Tylenol, ibuprofen)

Gas Ex: used for bloating and gas
Mylanta: used for upset stomach and indigestion
Peptol Bismol: for nausea and diarrhea
Pepcid: for indigestion and reflux
Amodium D: for diarrhea
Pedialyte or Gatorade: for hydration after diarrhea
Milk of Magnesia: for constipation
Bacitracin: for minor cuts and scrapes
Ice & heat packs: used for any minor aches, pains, swelling, and great for back pain
Biofreeze- cooling roll-on or gel for deep tissue pain
Arnica natural pain reliever- found in health food stores, pharmacy- great for muscle aches

I recommend cream Arnica over gel

Thermometer-digital: this helps detect any increase in body temperature, and can give us a heads up before health declines.

A low grade temperature can mean many things- depending on patient's medical history. If retaining fluid or congestion in lungs, it can easily lead to bronchitis or pneumonia. Daily monitoring is essential.

Always be sure to ask the patient's doctor if any allergies exist. Go over all routine OTC drugs and prescribed medications, as well.

CHAPTER 5

Meals and dietary needs

Meals and dietary needs are most important in keeping the patient alert, aware and fulfilled. The older we get, the more challenged we become, and our immune systems can be extremely fragile. Proper diets are always personalized for each particular patient according to their health and condition.

Certain patients require pureed foods due to poor swallowing reflexes, as well as thickened fluids (Hormel makes pre-packaged juice and water) which can be quite satisfying. Purees are very easy to prepare, and thickening powder ("thick-it", which can be found on Amazon.com) can be very helpful. I use "the bullet", mixer or a blender to puree, which is great for all pureed foods.

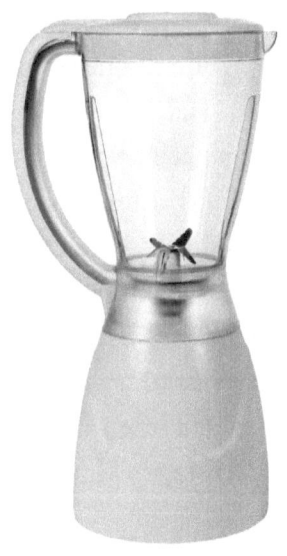

Remember, taste and smell are with us 'til the end! Creating a palatable meal brings joy and a positive outlook to one's future. Many elderly patients are no longer thirsty, therefore become dehydrated very easily. Keep track of fluids on a daily routine board. It is important to always have a container with fluid by their side, day and night. Constant reminders are necessary, and can help to keep them home and healthy. I have always tried to provide favorite juices or teas to help with hydration. Preparing food is a constant & making enough food is a good idea. Some patients can chew easily, so fresh vegetables are a perfect addition but only last a few days. When pureeing food, I make double batches & freeze for future use. Keep them eating & drinking to lift their spirits. It definitely works, so never give up! See more in Chapter 7!

Ask patients about their likes & dislikes, puddings, desserts, ice cream and breads can be very satisfying and nutritious. I usually add seasonings without salt to add to the flavor and entice eating. A routine is very important and creates balance within our body and soul. Be sure to constantly remind the caregivers to feed and hydrate them often. The stronger they are the easier it will be to stay healthy.

CHAPTER 6

Bathing

Bathing an unstable person is not easy, but extremely necessary for their future health and well-being. Showers are easiest with special chairs, so patients can be seated while aide uses hand-held sprayers to properly cleanse.

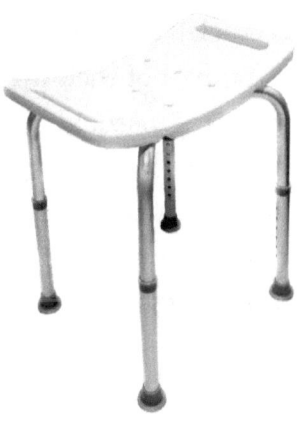

Handrails in and out of shower should be installed by a professional for safety.

As well as being clean, there are many products which can be used to prevent skin irritations and sores. When caring for sensitive and elderly patients, so many issues can become irreversible. Be sure to use barrier creams on private areas, or body parts on patients that are wheelchair bound or bed ridden, to avoid possible bed sores. Some examples of barrier creams that I would recommend are: ***"3M Cavilon durable barrier cream", "Soothe and cool moisture barrier ointment",*** found online, or others prescribed by a physician. If looking for a barrier cream in-store, a pharmacist can make helpful recommendations. One quick "go-to" would be ***"A &D" ointment.*** However, I don't recommend using a product with zinc, because it is difficult to remove. Something with a gel consistency is best. In an immune-challenged person, healing is crucial. Remember, daily cleansing should be an integral part of their lives.

Always consider using soap and shampoo products that are their favorites, or hypoallergenic. Make sure not to irritate delicate tissues or eyes.

A toilet commode fits over the existing toilet, and legs adjust for specific heights.

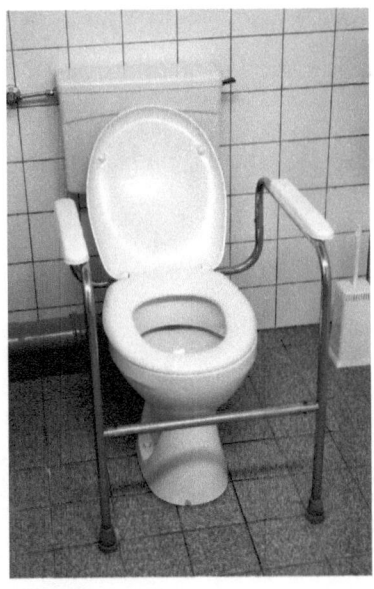

This helps when the patient cannot get on and off the traditional toilet due to back injury or weakness. The side arms on the commode enable them to lift up much easier and feel secure, as well.

Another item that I find helpful is flushable wipes. You can also purchase a container of baby wipes, and dispose of in the garbage. They are larger and easier to use in some cases. This enables the caregiver to wipe and clean the patient properly without tearing delicate tissue. At this time, barrier cream should be applied.

When caring for incontinence, all pull-ups should be checked and changed several times a day, due to rashes and sores that can occur when sitting in soiled undergarments. Once again, apply barrier cream (of course, using gloves at all times) after properly cleansing private areas. Always be sure to have a large supply of gloves, pull-ups, pads, and wipes for your patient.

CHAPTER 7

Housekeeping

Housekeeping and care for the home is another task not to be taken lightly. Many patients insist they can do it all, but as we know, simple errands, food shopping, and laundry can eliminate accidents on the outside, as well as in the home.

Keeping the house clean can prevent illnesses. Consider using non-latex gloves while preparing food and bathing, changing, etc. All glove sizes are available, so keeping the appropriate sizes of gloves on hand for yourself and aides is a good idea. Aides can work closely with the housekeepers, and can keep track of food shopping, and inventory of prepared meals. All foods should be monitored with dates on all containers. Check every day to be sure food is not spoiled. It's a good idea to purchase smaller storage bowls with lids for easy access and stacking in fridge.

We usually do cooking every few days, and make a double batch as to freeze extras. This makes it easier to always have their favorite meals on hand without running out.

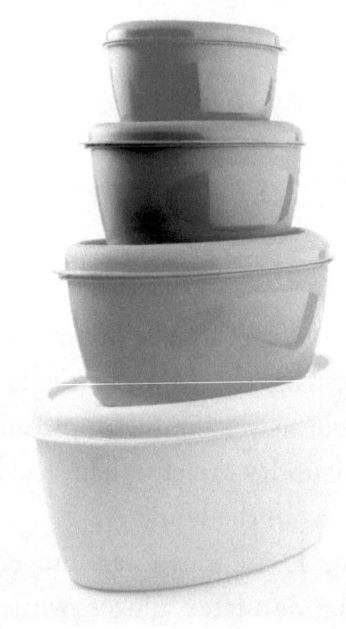

Seek out some hired help or volunteers to help with housekeeping, if possible. There are many young people out there looking for small jobs and very easy to hire. Volunteers can be found in many ways, for example, seniors are involved in churches, hospitals, etc. If you could find a few to do shopping, banking, and drives to medical appointments, this will help the family a great deal.

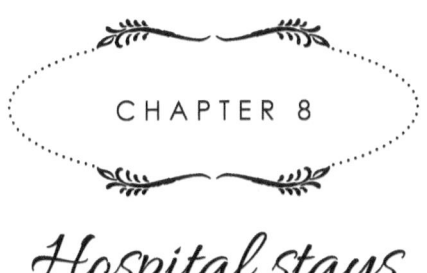

CHAPTER 8

Hospital stays

Hospital stays are unpredictable and it's a good idea to plan for events causing hospitalization. Most people have certain needs, and would like to have important items with them for any possible admission. Packing an overnight bag can save a lot of time and anguish on the patient's part, as well as the family or caregivers.

All bath and hygiene products, along with glasses, books, puzzles, etc., can be a lifesaver! Also, if they have a cell phone, remember to take along charger with phone. Being capable of any communication is a huge plus.

Most hospital visits convert to local nursing homes for some sort of rehabilitation. Be aware of choosing one by visiting before the need arises. For hospitals, as well as nursing homes, an advocate needs to be present to navigate the system. Leave name and numbers with doctors and staff, and ask to be contacted for updates and decisions for care. It can be a matter of survival!

Insurance info should be known and notated, for all benefits, and doctor visits, as well. It's important to keep all insurance, Medicare, and social security numbers in a wallet, and also listed in a journal. If they also have supplemental insurance, notify all doctors and hospitals.

Speak with the patient about their finances, and be aware of their financial situation. If they receive a social security check or pension, auto deposit can be arranged. Be prepared to pay bills while patient is hospitalized.

CHAPTER 9

Doctor's visits

Doctor's visits should be planned by one of the caregivers, so all important reports by given doctor can be explained to patient and aide. It's also a good idea to give the doctor a clear picture of the patient's current health. Even when they prefer their independence and privacy, in the end, you can provide much better care when all concerned are informed and prepared for care.

If you need more than one caregiver when traveling, plan ahead, so the patient can be mobilized in a wheelchair or with their walker. Again, ask the doctor what to expect, and how you can improve upon their quality of life.

Sometimes, exercise, naps, or communication with others can make a huge difference!

I recommend that the main advocate goes to the physician with the patient. With the patient's permission, you can obtain medical info as far as a list of prescriptions and all medical conditions you need to be aware of. Also, consider using the internet or books to help with any questions you may have.

Organize and list all important numbers and contacts! This master list is invaluable in order to keep patient and caregivers in touch. Patients feel reassurance simply by knowing help is just a phone call away.

Example:	Police	Taxi
	Fire	Pharmacy
	Family	Volunteers/Aides
	Friends	Local food store
	Electrician	Dentist
	Plumber	Doctors
	Heating	Ambulette service
	Repairman	
	Snow Removal	
	Gardener	

I usually list all caregivers and family numbers on the bottom of the main calendar, for quick reference. See list above when preparing your personalized list.

CHAPTER 10

Awareness

It's so important to be aware of the patient's needs, as well as illness versus wellness. Knowing the health history of the patient helps in knowing what to look for. Elderly patients have thinner skin and weaker bones. This makes them extremely sensitive to falls and skin tears. Consider buying bandages with paper tape-which will not tear skin upon removal. A minor trip and fall for an elderly person can be life-threatening.

Regular, routine (daily or weekly) body checks of the patient can be vital for their well-being. The purpose is to check for bedsores, lacerations, and rashcs. Bed sores can seriously affect the patient's mood, and can end up being fatal, if undetected and untreated. Prevention of sores is the best possible

route to go. Use of barrier creams is essential. ***see
examples of barrier creams in chapter 6***

Ask the patient questions, such as, "How's their
breathing, any pains?" The slightest change can be
huge in the life of an elder. The idea is to maintain
optimum mental and physical health. Try to be in
tune to any mood change or decline in appetite.
These can be a sign of an underlying problem.

At a certain age, we are no longer thirsty and do
not crave fluids. Therefore, dehydration can occur
very easily in the elderly. So, it is necessary to itemize
how much one drinks daily. ***see daily routine board
in Chapter 3.*** Signs of dehydration are noticeable in
the skin (becomes dry and flaky), and mouth appears
dry, with chapped lips.

CHAPTER 11

Activity

Planning a schedule for activity and exercise is as important as food intake. Moving them, walking, daily exercises, physical and speech therapy in many cases is the best way to improve health. It boosts mood, lowers risk of heart disease, diabetes, high blood pressure, and many other illnesses.

Daily routines are what most people lack, especially if someone is alone. Create regiment and watch them thrive! ***see board for activities in chapter 3.***

It should begin from the moment they awaken. Slow movement in stretching is essential, and it feels good too! While preparing for breakfast, a quick walk using the walker or cane can be a positive way to start the day. This can be part of the regiment before and after every meal. The more exercise, the better. Yoga

& light exercise designed for each particular person can be so relaxing for body & mind. Circulation is a huge part of their health, so increase movement whenever possible.

CHAPTER 12

Companionship

Being a caregiver is a difficult course, but there are many ways to receive the necessary help. Some people are used to being alone, so you need to slowly introduce them to an outsider. A companion can be a wonderful turning point. If you find someone who drives, they can plan outings, visits to friends or family, or a simple trip to the store. Creating normalcy is the goal.

Ads for students or retired persons are ideal for volunteers or paid companions.

Reading or listening to music from their era can create a positive outlook. Also, reading articles or books to them can help them feel connected to someone. I usually try to have the caregivers play a board or word game, or even cards, it helps them engage differently. Now they look forward to the companionship… remember the goal is to create quality in their life.

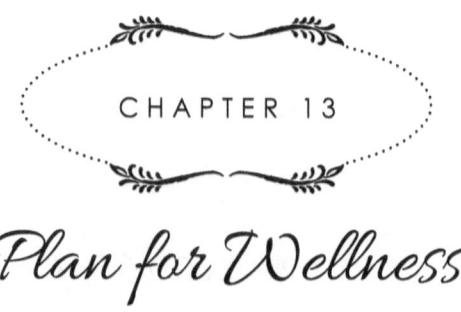

CHAPTER 13

Plan for Wellness

Emotional and mental health concerns can be a huge part of well-being. Balancing stress, depression, and anxiety and caring for their physical issues can be a challenge. I try to get as much information as possible from doctors and family members. As long as you are aware of their medical condition and have approval from the professionals for each particular case, you can begin to treat body, mind and soul.

I use many holistic modalities which include educating the caregivers first. If back pain is chronic, the use of heat pads and Arnica (natural pain reliever cream) is a soothing relief as well as using Bio Freeze roll on. Acupuncture and massage, if approved by the physician can be wonderful additions to their routines, creating relaxation and increased circulation.

I am a Reiki healer, which is energy work. Combining all of these holistic works, we can surely help raise immune systems and bring awareness of the connection between mind and body.

Music therapy can be used to heal from the inside out, mainly working on the heart, according to the Harvard Heart Letter.* It helps the recovery from a cardiac procedure, and can lower blood pressure. Coping with any illness is difficult enough for elders, so keep in mind- we want to soothe these delicate hearts.

Mental stimulation is part of the daily routine, ask which method they prefer. Puzzles, workbooks, board games, even simple game shows on TV, can improve their brain health, while increasing confidence. It is so important to stay focused on keeping them happy **every day**!

- **Footnote, Harvard Heart Letter**

CHAPTER 14

Checklists

Now that you have the basics laid out for you in this guide, I have compiled some handy checklists for family and caregivers to utilize.

Visit my website www.noplacelikehomebook.com for printable copies of these checklists and other valuable resources.

Checklist #1: For a family member:

o   Identify important financial information and familiarize yourself with the patient's assets

o   Know monthly income, and where it is coming from, list all income and expenses

o   Know medical history and doctors' contact numbers

o   Know who to call and how to care for repairs and home maintenance

o   Research insurance, whether it be Medicare, Medicaid, or supplemental coverage

o   Obtain copies of Social Security cards, medical coverage, Veteran benefits, if applicable, life insurance & retirement benefits

o   Identify patient's ability to manage finances themselves, or look for the signs that patient needs assistance with managing finances

o   Acquire power of attorney for person closest to the decision making, whether it be financial or medical

o   Final arrangements: know person's wishes, such as, organ donor, final will, and burial plans

<u>Checklist #2: For caregivers</u>

o Stay on top of patient's daily needs

o Check daily routine board

o Appoint one main caregiver to distribute and keep track of patient's daily health and medications

o Prepare fresh foods (puree if necessary) according to patients' needs and desires

o Maintain patient's personal hygiene including laundry and bedding

o Maintain clean home, including bathrooms and kitchens

o Plan to engage patient in exercise, reading, or games

o Make necessary appointments on behalf of patient's needs, such as: doctors, hair, personal needs

o Check and double check for safe environment (identify possible tripping hazards, or fall risks)

Checklist #3: Blank checklists

(to be used for caregivers or family members to utilize additionally)

o

o

o

o

o

o

o

o

o

o

o

o

o

o

o

o

o

o

o

o

o

o

o

<u>Blank Checklist</u>

o

o

o

o

o

o

o

o

o

o

o

o

o

o

o

o

o

o

o

o

o

o

o

o

o

o

o

o

About the Author

Joyce Greene has been involved in caregiving most of her life. Through caring for her family members, especially her mother, she taught herself to navigate the eldercare system. Joyce resides in Westchester County, N.Y. with her husband, David, and of course, her mother. Joyce is the practice director at Scarsdale Dental Spa and Wellness, where she works with her husband, Dr. Greene. Their state of the art dental practice caters to clientele looking for a tranquil and peaceful environment, which enables their patients to overcome dental phobias.

She is available for phone consultations, please email for appointments at joyce@joycegreene.com or visit our web site www.noplacelikehomebook.com